Index

1

Introduction

There's no universal formula to achieving success in life, but a few essential guidelines are to remember. The first is always to place your success first. Do not place yourself under pressure to do anything which doesn't bring you joy or aid you in reaching your objectives. Thirdly, stay focused. Don't be apathetic about your goals or dreams.

Also, surround yourself with positive people who will be there for you in achieving your objectives. You can take many things to increase your odds of success in your life when you have a small penis. You can make informed decisions, make good choices, establish good habits, and surround yourself with positive people. But what is most crucial could be done is to be clear about the goals you wish to reach and then put in the effort to get them.

There are many things that people wish they had known about how to achieve success on the path of life. The fact is that there's no universally applicable solution. However, there are a handful of essential rules that can aid you in achieving success in every aspect of your daily life. In the first place, you must remain persevering.

If you're looking for something, pursue it with your heart, soul, and determination. Don't let go of your goals or dreams, even if they appear difficult initially.

The culture has taught us to think that having a small size penis is a negative issue and that we should feel ashamed of it. The reality is that there are plenty of successful men in the world who have a small penis and couldn't care less. They just learned to deal with it.

Thanks to this book you will be able to overcome your fears and to understand the real advantages of having a small penis. You will learn the best strategies to be successful in sex and to be comfortable with your penis regardless the size; you will learn that "dimensions" it's just a matter of perspective.

2

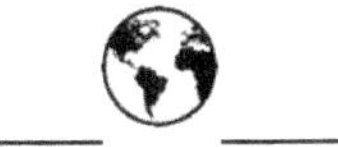

The Average Penis Size Around The Globe

Each man has his expectations regarding their male organ size, but does the size of an individual's body part correlate with the size of the other male organs across the globe? The penises of men worldwide are bigger than the penises of North American men. This is probably due to cultural influences but might not reflect the reality of all males.

There isn't a single answer to this question since the size of a man's body varies based on where you live and the culture. The median length of men's female genitals was 6.5 inches across and 4.7 inches. Men's measurements from six nations: Brazil, Canada, France, Germany, Italy, and the United States. The size of a man's average across the globe varies based on the location. Like Africa, the average penis size is relatively small in some areas.

In contrast, the other hand, in North America and Europe, the penis size average is much larger. The reason for this is that there are a variety of reasons. One explanation is that cultural distinctions play an essential role in what is thought to be an adequate man's size. In addition, genetic factors affect the size of a man's body.

If you've ever thought about what your penis's size is compared to others in regards to size, you're not all on your own. Men are always curious to see how their penises are compared to average. However, this curiosity may lead to an utterly overwhelming obsession and anxiety about the size of your penis. This can lead to unhealthy and sometimes unneeded concerns, mainly since most men who believe their penises aren't big enough are normal-sized men.

What's the typical size of a penis? A study of more than 15,000 males revealed an average length of 3.6 inches and the flaccid's average circumference (girth) in the range of 3.7 inches. When they were erect, the penises measured the average that was 5.1 inches, and the average circumference was 4.5 inches.

It's possible that this is not exactly what you were expecting. In a society where we have long associated big penises with power, virility, and masculinity, The notion that big penises are commonplace is widely accepted. In the past, males from across the globe have utilized several unwise methods to grow in size their penises.

The Cholomec tribe from Peru and Sadhus males from India put weights on their penises to lengthen them. Then in Brazil, Topinama tribe members allowed poisonous snakes to bite their penises and expand their Size and Size by expanding.

Today, males who aren't satisfied by the shape of their genitals may consider stretching techniques for their penises, such as "jelqing" (which may have limited or only temporary effects at most), or even think about surgery if their penises are perfectly average in dimensions.

Some have suggested that porn can contribute to unfounded expectations regarding the size of the penis and the notion in the notion that the size of the penis is the primary aspect in determining an intimate partner's satisfaction and satisfaction. Numerous studies have shown that most male-female partners don't emphasize the shape that their penises are. A study of females who were sexually active revealed that 77% of women surveyed found the size of their partner's penises was not important (55 percent) or insignificant (22 percent). Additionally, in a study of more than 52,000 people, around 83% of women stated that they were satisfied with their partners' penis length, and only 55% of males were happy.

Little research has been conducted regarding the importance of bisexual and gay men, considering how big their penises are. One study on the subject revealed that men with female sexual companions have a better notion of the actual size of their penis than those who have only female partners because of their higher and more intimate interaction with other penises.

Because the average size of the penis is smaller and less important to partners than men think and it's likely that men's worries oversize are untrue. However, if you notice that your penis is frequently causing anxiety or discomfort, consult your physician or therapist about the issue.

The perennial question now has a scientific answer of 13.12 centimeters (5.16 inches) in length when upright and 11.66cm (4.6 inches) around, following an analysis of over 15,000 penises from around the globe. In a swollen state, it was discovered that the penis of a typical male is 9.16cm (3.6 inches) in length. It also is girth-wise 9.31cm (3.7 inches).

Men are too anxious about the size of their penis to forget about it. These numbers will reassure the large majority of men that the size of their penis is in the normal range, as results of studies in which a specialist examined participants.

The team used the numbers gathered to design an illustration that doctors could employ in counseling men suffering from "small penis anxiety."

In extreme instances, the men could suffer from body dysmorphic disorders - an uncontrollable psychological disorder that can cause an obsession with antisocial behavior or depression. It can also lead to suicide. In the real world, the reality is that just 2.28 percent of the male population has an abnormally small penis, as per the study, and an identical percentage has an unusually large one.

The participants in the study were men aged between 17 and 91 years old who were able to measure their penises in studies previously published and carried out throughout Europe, Asia, Africa, and the United States.

The team could not find evidence of differences in penis size related to race, even though the majority of those who participated are of European and Middle Eastern descent, and a comprehensive comparison was not able to be drawn.

Researchers did not find any evidence of a significant correlation between a man's size of his feet and the size of his manhood. They acknowledged that their findings could be somewhat biased because males willing to undergo a medical exam might be more confident about their penis size than the general population.

It's amazing how nearly every person on Earth has the exact dimensions of their penis right to the millimeter. Knowing your sexual measurements is a fundamental personal fact alongside your weight, height, and blood type. A post-Pornhub society does have certain disadvantages (and this isn't just referring to the baffling growth in popularity of "step porn"). Because the infamously sensationalized kind of adult entertainment demands an element of, let's say, cinematic style - that many believe to be the norm.

Never have there been more confusion over the typical size of the penis in every aspect, including the typical length of an erect penis to the general dimensions of penises. Nearly 45 percent of men think that they have a small penis. The testicles and the penis in humans tend to stop growing when you reach the age of 18 (towards the end of the puberty stage).

Once you reach 18, you're left with what you have unless you undergo any medical intervention, whether extracurricular or not (more on this later). The average size of a man's body across the globe is very different. In certain parts of the globe, males have large penises. However, in other regions around the globe, the size of the penis is considered to be small. Below are the five most important facts regarding male size across the globe:

1. In Africa, the size of the penis can be considered huge. An average African man is a size for penis of 13 inches.

2. Asia is the continent with the smallest average penis size, 8 inches.

How Big Is The Average Size Of A Penis?

For a long time, studies relied on self-reporting being prone to bias from volunteers and perceptions about social likability. This affected the quality of the data collection. It's not easy to admit that they're using light equipment, and even the best operator have had to provide more sizzle by offering a steak. Historically, the larger size of the penis is considered more attractive. The size of the penis is a frequent cause of stress for males due to unrealistic expectations of what's normal that are pushed by porn and media. A surprising number of males worry about whether their penis is enough.

To aid the people suffering from Body Dysmorphic Disorder and males who feel worried about their dick size, the complete research available on penis size and drawn from 20 studies involving more than 15,500 people. Researchers determined that the median penis size -based on the data of over 15500 men, measured 3.6 millimeters (9.16 centimeters) when flaccid and 5.2 (13.12 centimeters) inches when standing up.

The study findings are a comfort to men of all ages as it confirms that the "six inches" average that's frequently proclaimed in the conversations in the media or on the street isn't the real size of a penis.

3

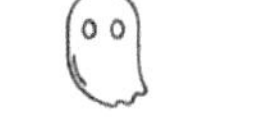

How Do You Overcome Fears About A Small Penis

The data could prove useful in reassured men concerned about their weight. However, it can also sabotage those who believe they are unusually wealthy. Doctors could utilize the graph to assist men in choosing the right condom for their needs.

We have one small request. Millions of people turn to the Guardian for honest and independent daily news. Readers across 180 countries across the globe are now financially supporting us. We believe that everyone should access information based on credibility and trustworthiness based on truth, science, and analysis.

We decided to make our content available to everyone regardless of their location or the amount they can spend. This allows more people to be more informed, united, and motivated to take action. In these turbulent times, an honest global news organization such as the Guardian is vital. We don't have shareholders or billionaire owners, so our reporting is not influenced by any political or commercial influence, making us unique.

It's never been more vital; our independence enables us to investigate without fear and challenge those in power. Regardless of the size of his penis, every man is worried that his penis is too big. You should be aware of the size of your penis and what you can do if you're concerned that your penis is bigger than "normal."

1. The Numbers

We'll start by talking about pure numbers. It's not easy to figure out the exact size of the penis because of various factors, such as reporting bias and cultural differences. However, the latest comprehensive study found that the median is just over 5 inches when in a straight position. 5.2 inches, to be precise. Most of my clients think that six or seven inches are the norm; however, that's not the reality.

2. Penis Size Doesn't Affect Pleasure

Here's the good news how big your penis doesn't impact the pleasure you're capable of experiencing. A bigger penis does not make you feel more comfortable during sexual activity. Contrary to what those nervous thoughts that lurk in your head may tell you that the size of your penis has minimal impact on how much pleasure your partner can be capable of experiencing.

If you're sleeping with women, the dimensions of your penis might not be as crucial as you think since it's not the most enjoyable sexual experience for females. Most nerve endings found in female genitals are concentrated on the clitoris. There are only a few nerve endings within the vaginal canal, and there's no scientifically-based tally of the vaginal canal's nerve endings. The nerves that the vagina has are located in the outermost third of the vagina. This means that deeper penetration isn't able to bring more enjoyment.

Perforation isn't the most enjoyable activity for women because it's not a great source of sensations in the clitoral area. In reality, 70 to 80 percent of women don't get to gas by merely piercing. Women can feel subtle distinctions between larger and smaller penises, but this is more about satisfaction. A larger penis isn't doing a much better job of stimulating the clitoral area as a smaller penis does.

If you are a man who sleeps with men and is the ever-penetrating partner in intimate sex, A smaller penis can be preferable. The rectum cannot stretch the way vaginas are; therefore, a smaller penis feels better than one with a bigger size.

Some prefer a larger-than-average penis. However, the size of the penis isn't an issue for most people. If you're worried about the shape of your penis, think about being in the other aspect of the problem.

Would you ditch your lover just due to its size? Or her genitals? or her breasts? or his penis? I doubt it.

I'm willing to wager that you view your partner as an entire human being, not just a collection of parts. Your partner should be able to perceive you similarly.

3. Sometimes It's About More Than Just Your Penis

For some men, anxiety over the size of their penis is a sign of an anxiety disorder that is more fundamental. If you are worried about the size of your penis every day or if your anxiety level appears to be excessive, you might want to concentrate on your daily anxiety control.

The advice for managing anxiety that I usually recommend is to be mindful. I enjoy using Headspace as it shows you how to be more mindful. It provides simple explanations that are easy to grasp. Headspace offers an introduction series you can test at no cost.

If you are satisfied, you can sign up for a small fee per month for additional series that cover a variety of subjects. In particular, you might like to look into their series on anxiety management. Many of my customers (especially male clients who have problems with performance) find this course extremely beneficial.

If you are experiencing penis size anxiety, then you might want to consider taking the time to take a short (or long-term) break from watching.

It's easy to forget that porn is supposed to entertain, and porn performers must have huge penises. If you're seeing massive penises regularly, it's not difficult to get a different view about the definition of "normal."

I've dealt with many clients who torture themselves with web-based research about the size of their penis. It could be how you came across this post!

Such research is not beneficial and often makes anxiety more severe. It is possible to install an extension for your browser to your computer to stop you from performing these search results. You can also restrict yourself from penis-sized websites and forums you usually browse. There's no reason to feel embarrassed or embarrassed for having a tiny penis. There are plenty of people who have a smaller member and still succeed in their lives.

4

Advantages Of Having A Small Penis

To provide an innocent analogy for an incredibly innocent action - it's your handwriting that counts more than the thickness of your pencil. Does size matter? The question has been around from the beginning of time with many manhood-related opinions. While a big penis may be impressive to boast about, it doesn't guarantee an enjoyable experience for your loved one unless you can perform the right act.

Anyone who has been making small penis jokes should listen to this! There are numerous benefits to having a small than average penis since they don't depend on their dicks to offer their friends the thigh-curling smooch, but they will look for other ways to make the game more interesting.

Human nature has a belief that "more is better." As men are obsessed with women's breasts or the shape of their asses and shapes, some women are obsessed with the size of the penis of their partners.

Are you looking to destroy the self-esteem of a man? Laugh while pointing at his penis as the man is dressed before you. A tiny penis is usually the Source of many jokes, and many men want that they are associated with a bigger model rather than a smaller one.

However, as has been widely said, skillful and good care for your penis is far more crucial in terms of satisfaction with sexual pleasure than the size of the penis. However, if there is nothing else but a physical appearance, it leaves men wanting to be branded for having a small penis. There are benefits of having a smaller large endowment.

1. **Lowered Expectations**

One of the main benefits of a smaller penis is that expectations are reduced. Many people believe that a large penis is going to mean great sex. However, that's not the case in all cases. The time between the moment of penetration to ejaculation is about 3 minutes.

That applies regardless of size. If your penis is larger, most women expect more but are disappointed. When they have a tiny penis, they aren't able to make high expectations, but they could be amazed at how effective their partner is in wooing them.

2. **Small Penises Suit Long-Term Relationships Just Fine**

A study from 2014 found that, when it comes to one-night dates, the size can be an issue. However, it also discovered that girth, not length is the most significant measurement.

The reason is the fact that the enjoyment derived from a penis-in-vagina (PIV) one-night affair generally is due to the level of intensity (that's the code word for the desire to get beat up); however, the sex of a long-term relationship benefits from a deeper understanding of the partner's preferences and likes. If you're in a relationship that includes using a penis, it is necessary to be patient.

It has a good understanding of the appropriate position, making it more suitable for an ongoing relationship in which emotional and personal feelings also play a role.

Even when making love, there is a lot you can do to ensure that your partner enjoys the experience. This generally involves being romantic, making time for foreplay, and including sufficient clitoral stimulation."

Only a small percentage of women orgasm from stimulation of the cervix. For most women, size] probably doesn't have any significance. It's likely to be equally great in the majority of instances.

3. More Care

In reality, an individual with a smaller penis is a remarkable lover. It's not uncommon for a modestly enthused man to be determined to prove that it is indeed an ability that is more important than the size. This is why the man may be more likely to engage in intense foreplay, try different postures, or take time to understand his partner's desires and wants. This doesn't mean that a man with an enormous penis would not perform this, but smaller penis men tend to be more likely to do it.

4. Better Condom Fit

Men with larger penises have complained that condoms aren't tight or do not suit properly. One of the advantages of having a small penis is the ease of finding a condom suitable for your needs - that is essential not just for comfort but also to reduce the possibility for the condom to break during sexual activity.

Are there negatives to having a tiny penis? Sure. However, they are mentioned all the time that men overlook certain advantages. Whatever the size of their bodies, they must appreciate what they have and think about how they can best utilize it.

The benefits are good regardless of whether you have an insignificant penis, medium or large one. Penises of all sizes can benefit from the daily application of a top-quality penis health cream, Man Oil, which has been clinically proven to be gentle and safe for the skin.

The most effective creams will contain several vitamins, like B5. Also called pantothenic acid, vitamin B5 is an essential nutrient needed to regulate cell metabolism and maintain healthy tissues. Penis skin is prettier and more appealing when the skin is moisturized (so pick a cream with Shea butter and Vitamin E) and if it can absorb lots of vitamin A (found in many creams) and is anti-aging and has blemish-fighting properties.

5. Circumcision Can Change How A Penis Is Perceived

While circumcision is very popular within America, circumcision is a popular choice in the United States. In other countries (aside from the people who undergo circumcision due to religious reasons), it's not as popular.

The benefits and disadvantages of circumcision are a constant debate, especially when discussing penis size or at least concerning appearance will have an impact. Circumcision is the removal of the foreskin, leaving the 'glans' exposed.

When flaccid, an uncircumcised penis could appear smaller than one that isn't due to the absence of the additional layer of tissue covering the glans. When it is erect, the foreskin shrinks and becomes virtually invisible, and so in terms of size, there's no discernible difference in how the penis appears."

Although it would be fantastic to give men the option of having their circumcision or not, especially considering the number of nerves destroyed by getting rid of the skin of the foreskin, this isn't the norm.

6. You Can Still Reach All Her Pleasure Points

The reason people believe they require a "big one" to be comfortable in bed, we will not know. The clitoris is a woman's most desirable pleasure point situated outside the vagina. A woman's G-spot lies only a few inches within. This means that even the smallest women can go to a delightful town.

Approximately 75% of women do not orgasm from vaginal penetration alone, no matter how large is the penis. This is among the many reasons I urge women to expand their definition of sex to include more than traditional sexual relations. Learn about your oral and digital abilities, play with sex toys, add sexually explicit massages and sexy conversations, and take advantage of your bedtime.

7. Bigger Doesn't Mean Better

There are no studies demonstrating that women feel more content with wealthy men. It's because not all men with big johnsons can utilize it to their advantage with any ability. Concentrate on the primary occasion, guys. You cannot change your size.

However, you can increase your skills. If you're not confident in your ability to push her to the edge, Try different positions, and think about introducing certain sex toys to the mix. Ask her whether she'd like to use these toys. Some women are uncomfortable when they ask their partners to use a vibrator or dildo, although they could be using them when doing masturbation.

8. It Is Easier To Learn For Both Anal And Oral Beginners

A few women would claim they prefer big dicks; however, we all know very few have had to contend with the size of a 10-inch monster in their tummies. Even the most experienced porn stars admit that they prefer the normal size penis for their private lives. The small size of the penis was a benefit in the past when my partner initially tried an anal or orally.

It's still an advantage for those who want to test an innovative technique. It's easier to confront a smaller foe even if it has the same thing as the monster. It is possible to go to the bottom without fearing the gag reflex, and I can go toe-deep in their stomachs without the anxiety of a tissue rupture or prolapse. It's a win-win...

9. Master Some Techniques

If you're a man with a smaller penis, you can learn ways to impress your loved one. The trick is to satisfy her needs and make her eyes spin like the game, with her mouth wide in a plea for air and her body shaking like an 11-scale earthquake (or his or hers, if you prefer males).

To get that legendary orgasm, you don't have to rely on your penis. You have to employ all the tools you have at your disposal. Toys, fingers, tongue massages, oils, candles, and kinks are a good way to please your lover and require you to master new techniques.

The tricks don't just apply to sexual tricks as they also include education about her erogenous body parts, dislikes or likes, and triggers for orgasm. Also, you must be educated about your body - those triggers you use, the kinks in your body, and your preferences. It is a process of practice, building stamina, and, most importantly, it requires communication.

5

★★★★★

How To Be Successful In Sex With A Small Penis - For Man and Woman

This is why it's so funny that so many men think larger is better for penis size. When fully in a straight position, an average penis measures 5.2 inches in length. In the same study, 90% of men have a penis between 4 to 6.3 inches when they are erect.

However, if you're among the remaining 10% (because you're bigger or smaller), a few different sexual tips and techniques will provide the enjoyment that you and your companions want. This doesn't mean that you shouldn't be able to enjoy mind-blowing sexual sex. However, you need to be aware of making the most of the sex you have in your favor.

A man's ability to give a woman pleasure and even orgasm doesn't depend on penis size. Hands, mouths, toys, and mouths are all great sources of pleasure that males can depend on. There are ways to alter sex postures to be more comfortable, depending on the size of your body.

For help in identifying the best moves and tactics that can ensure that you and your partner always want to return to the bed, the most effective ways to experience amazing experiences even when you're not as wealthy. These suggestions will bring your sex experience to the next level and make it more fulfilling.

1. Communicate

Keeping the communication lines open is crucial if you're insecure about your capacity to please your spouse. "Partners need to communicate about many aspects of their sexual relationship. Pleasuring that you are in love isn't an automatic thing, but rather it is something that two individuals teach one another.

Women may require an exact stimulation method to get their orgasm, while a male may require a particular method of being slapped to have a sexual erection. Similar to that, the size of the penis of a male could be the subject of conversations.

People who love one another will discuss the subject with respect and openness. They will talk about ways to overcome the issue and work together to discover ways to enhance happiness for both partners.

2. Try Rear Entry

After you've addressed any issues with your spouse, it's time to get into the fun part of experimenting and figuring out the best solution for you! A position that experts endorse will surely take the lady and you on an exciting adventure: the doggy. Certain postures increase friction and feel. For instance, a 'doggy' style with the man at the back, and the female sitting on her knees in front of him, typically gives women a sensation of intersex, particularly if she tucks her thighs in.

Fleming agrees that having a woman squeeze her legs together will make sexual intimacy more enjoyable for both partners. Rear entry is a good position for smaller men because it can allow him to reach their G-spot, which is about 3-inches inside the anterior vaginal wall."

3. Use Props

For men who have a smaller penis, sexual sex is about finding the most effective angles. Fleming says. "Utilize your surroundings furniture, furniture, and other props to determine the most suitable angles and the depth of penetration suitable for the two of you. When you're standing doggy, consider putting your hands on chairs; pillows under the hips, while she's at the lower part of the body, can assist in getting deeper into a "full" feeling many women are looking at.

That is why women mostly feel their best when they touch their clitoris. Try putting a small vibration on her clitoris as you push to increase pleasure and sensation. As she gets more excited, her vaginal walls are tighter, making sex pleasant for you.

4. Skip The Lube

One thing you should not have in your sex kit? Lube. "If she's already lubricated, you don't need to add any more. A little friction can enhance the sensation," explains Fleming. Be aware that if she's dry, the sensation of penetration can be uncomfortable regardless of the size. You'll need to concentrate on activating her and making her feel better before you begin grinding and bouncing.

5. Have Her Put Her Legs Up

If deepening your relationship with her is something you are looking for, ask her to place her legs across your shoulders while in the posture of a missionary. This will give you more pleasure and enjoyment. It is also possible to have her lie down with her back against the side of your couch or bed and her legs straight up. When you enter her in this position, it can maximize what you've got. You want vaginal access without the obstruction of other body parts.

6. Let Her Climb On Top

Another option to try is woman-on-top. It's one of the best strategies for a guy with a smaller penis, as it allows the woman to maximize her partner's length and position him in a way that feels good to her. It can also give the person (or your partner!) the power to activate her clitoris. This is typically required to get that huge O. To ensure you don't slip out when playing dirty, let her rock and grind against your body instead of bouncing between the sides.

7. Extend Foreplay

Whatever position you're tempted to take, be aware that the length of your foreplay can make sexual intimacy more enjoyable for both you and your partner, not just as it creates arousal that is the key to having more intense orgasms. If you're worried about your weight or your ability to impress a woman by playing (and getting her to gasp) before taking it to the next level will help ease the pressure off of the main event.

8. Don't Stress

The first thing to note is that having a smaller penis isn't big. There's a piece of interesting information that will bring you and many of the less hefty guys on the market at peace: most nerve endings within the vaginal canal are located in the third outer. So long as you get the outer third filled (which most penises do), you'll receive ample stimulation.

Also, penetration isn't the primary thing for many women. Many women prefer sexual stimulation via oral or by hand more. Moreover, most women aren't able to orgasm due to the vaginal area alone.

9. Obey The Golden Rule

If the guy you're dating mentions subtly that his penis size is huge, please do not be negative! Remember your Golden Rule in the back of your thoughts. I'm sure that, at the very least, one area of your body makes you feel uneasy, So think of the way you'd like to be treated if you were to ask whether your thighs were too flapping or your thighs too big. If he's pushing or squirts, tell him, "I like how our bodies fit together" or "I believe we share an abundance of chemistry. I'm paying more focus on that than everything else.

10. Find Your Best Positions

If you're ever having a sexual encounter with a stranger, it is crucial to determine the appropriate positions for your body. This wrote about the top positions for men more petite.

It is generally recommended to look for positions that allow you to keep your legs in the right position to maintain a snug shape.

It is also beneficial to choose positions where your crotches are kept close. (For instance, standing sex positions can be difficult because there is a tendency to be a significant amount of space between your bodies.

11. Work Your Kegels

Keeping those PC muscles in good shape will help keep the proper alignment during your intercourse. Your PC muscles form a hammock across your pelvis. They perform different functions and can also aid in causing your vaginal walls to contract and feel more firm. As with any muscle in your body, exercises can make them stronger.

When you next have to pee, try to stop peeing before your bladder has been empty. You'll feel the internal "pulling up" type of sensation. Try 10 sets of quick pulses and 10 repetitions of more extended holds each day. When you're with your partner, you can try to squeeze your PC muscles as your partner smacks your body.

A bonus is that a stronger PC has been associated with the greater orgasmic output!

12. Consider Using Less Lube

If you've read one of my other posts on sexual relations, you've probably noticed that I'm a huge advocate of lube. However, this is one of the few instances where I'm not recommending excessive lube use. If you're very wet, it might appear like the lube is slipping within you too much.

If you're using lubricant, make sure you use an amount of dime-sized or less. Have him take them out if you think things are slippery, even without other lubricants. Try a handshake for about 15 minutes. Your hands will remove some of the lubricants, and you'll have additional friction after you resume conversations.

13. Add More Clitoral Stimulation

As I said earlier, the third outermost region of vaginal canals is the most vital part. However, this area's number of nerve endings is abysmal compared to the number of nerve endings found in the clitoris. Check out my earlier articles for advice for focusing more attention on oral sex and manual stimulation. Try increasing the clitoral stimulation you experience during your intercourse with your clitoris and having him do it or even having someone else play with the toy.

14. Experiment With Anal

One of the advantages of dating a guy who has a smaller penis is that anal sex is enjoyable! Many women say that anal sex can be painful for men who are bigger than average However, you're much less likely to experience this issue. This could be the ideal moment to begin exploring the pleasures of anal.

15. Use Toys

If you and this person can stay together for a few months and are an enthusiast of intense penetration, tools are available. I wouldn't suggest making these suggestions until you both have an established relationship.

If you are a girl, concentrate more on the possibility that you'd like to explore new ideas instead of focusing on the issue of being "too small." You could try putting him onto a penis sleeve or an extender. You can also make him enter your body by using a vibrator. Also, you can consider making him use the strap-on dildo. You can even aim for double penetration!

16. Include Other Body Components

Sexual intimacy isn't just about the penis rubbing the vagina. When it's a complete body experience, it's more enjoyable. Inviting all your muscles to join in will boost arousal and help your body feel "filled up" if he's smaller.

Grip his body by squeezing your thighs together and tightening your stomach. Don't forget the other good-for-you areas beyond the penis. "Gently rub his scrotum or massage the area between the scrotum and anus. The coccyx, also known as the backbone of the tail, is also stuffed with nerve endings.

Therefore, applying gentle pressure every time he's standing on top of it can make all the difference.

17. Simply Breathe

Many women breathe rapidly in sex, and the breath is held as they're about to get their sex. Do not do this! It is possible to intensify the sensation of your orgasm and let it last for a long and deliciously enjoyable time by controlling your breathing. It's a lot more difficult to achieve than it is; however, as you get more focused, concentrate on breathing slowly and deeply and resist the urge not to breathe.

In this way, you'll be able to allow the tension to increase and construct until you can help but feel an exhilarating scream that Christian Grey would be proud of.

18. Try A New Routine

In a recent study on the sexual preferences of married couples, almost 30% of women admitted that they would like their husbands to last longer. In reality, you're the one who can make your wish come true. All you need to do is alter your routine.

Men's testosterone levels are highest at night, so they're ready for early a.m. and may remain longer during the morning nookie sex. A majority of couples will have sexual encounters in the evening before hitting the hay.

However, when you're exhausted from work, children, and all the day's stresses, you don't have plenty of fuel to trip to a pleasant city. Do a quick morning session and keep a sweet smile throughout the day.

6

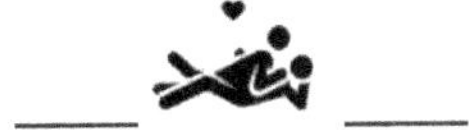

The Best Sex Position For Men With A Small Penis

Our society is based on a culture that gives arbitrary and unjust significance to men's penis. If you ask your average person what they think the average penis size is, they'd probably tell you six, six-and-a-half, or even seven inches. This is a subject that has plenty of confusion and misinformation around.

The typical size of a penis is five to five and an inch erect and straight. In this way, it's difficult to remove a feeling of genital insecurity in the mind of a man with a modestly wealthy background. It's worth noting that women aren't concerned: A survey of 1100 Cosmopolitan subscribers (96 percent who were identified as female) found that 89 percent of them were not concerned about the size of their partner's gift.

This is probably because most women realize that the size of the penis isn't the main aspect of sexual pleasure. It's all about finding the best posture or movement to induce an orgasm.

However, if your guy is concerned about slippage or has been there IRL, Here are six options that are guaranteed to please. It's a way to shame people and reinforce the notion that those with bigger penises (and everyone who has the penises) appear to have more masculinity than the rest of us. The popularity of mainstream porn and the shocking deficiency of sex education across the US certainly does not aid in this.

If there's no proper sexual education, small penis jokes are broken in every comedy and sitcom, and the only penises you'll see are 8-inch wangs on porn. what are you to be taught anything other than "size matters?"

I'm not saying that this is a lie. I'm not saying this to make myself sound more positive about my body or help any person feel better. These are factual statements. Research has consistently demonstrated that when it comes down to penis size, females (and women who have vaginas) generally place the length of the penis very low in their list of positive characteristics of a penis.

Girth is the one that tops the list, and biologically, this is logical. The vagina is home to several nerve endings that feel pressure. Still, only a handful of nerve endings that are touch sensitive and, therefore, pressure and the sensation of fullness make the biggest distinction in vaginal pleasure. Consider that up to one in five women suffers from painful sexual contact (for various motives).

The canal for the vagina measures between 3 and 6 inches in length and one up to 2.5 millimeters wide (when not stimulated). This makes it evident that larger doesn't mean better, especially for the receiving person.

Additionally, female orgasm is not often achieved by only penetration. Most clitoris-owners experience orgasms via external clitoral stimulation. This means that the penis doesn't play a role in female orgasm.

Whether big or small, if you're a master of oral sex or hand sexuality skills, it won't matter what you're doing on the ground. The standard length of the penis measured 5.16 inches. If your penis is just short of the benchmark and you're statistically tinier than average. Most people find it not an issue.

Research has revealed that women don't care too much about their size; according to the old saying that it's not how big the waves are but the movement of the ocean that's important. You'll be in good condition if you know the most effective sex postures for men with a smaller penis and a small penis.

However, if you've got a smaller than average penis, you may be worried about it. Some men mistake comparing themselves to porn stars--the Olympic athletes of sex-- that aren't realistic. In my therapeutic experience, most women do not talk about wanting a man with a big penis. They talk about wanting a man who is good in bed.

That means someone is communicative, takes his time, and is attentive to her needs. Furthermore, if you can master the system, it is possible to use the smaller size of your penis for your benefit. "Anecdotally, I've heard that men with small penises are better in bed because they make more effort. If you're less than rich, Here are a few sex roles to maximize the value for your money (pun not intended).

1. Doggie Style

If you have a little penis, "as a general rule, you want to go for any position that facilitates deep penetration so that you can utilize the entire length of your shaft. This is the reason why Doggie Style is a great choice. "It's not difficult and gives you a fantastic rear-view and allows you to extend your reach to give her extra stimulation to the clitoral.

You can control the speed and the pattern of your thrusts to ensure maximum enjoyment and penetration.

2. Face-Off

This is the ideal position for those with a slim penis, as it's more focused on "in and out" penetration it's more of "wiggling" around while you're in your partner's presence. It also permits kissing or nipple play as well as excessive petting.

It's possible to consider wearing the ring of a vibrating cock when you are in this position. If you deep thrust with a vibrating ring, you'll be providing intense clitoral stimulation with your thrusts, compensating for the lack of cervical stimulation.

3. The Little Dipper

To perform The Little Dipper, your partner can use a couch, bed, or chair to lift their body on top of you. Then, you insert the penis of your partner's anus or vagina, depending on how you feel the most comfortable! If you've done it correctly, it should form a T-shaped pattern.

This position allows deep penetration and the ability to access stimulating the clitoral area easily. The clitoris is the powerhouse of female pleasure. The vagina has far fewer nerve endings than the clitoris, which is only intermittently stimulated during most standard intercourse positions. That's why the positions that permit deeper vaginal penetration are perfect for women with less slender penis.

4. Cowgirl

There are a variety of cowgirl styles that you can look over here. It's hard to pick the best one for those who have a smaller penis as it's all about how small your penis is and its angle. Check if your regular cowgirl is performing the task. If not, consider switching to a squatting cowgirl that permits deep penetration, manual clitoral stimulation, and G-spot stimulation.

5. Stand and Deliver

Also called The Bicycle, Stand and Deliver provides a surprisingly deep reach. You stand at the edge of your desk or bed while your partner reclines and lifts their legs to their chests. Their knees are bent like they're performing the "bicycling" exercise. After that, they should grasp their ankles and walk into them. Another position permits deep penetration as well as manual clitoral stimulation.

6. Elevated Reverse Cowgirl

Elevated reverse cowgirl is an alteration to the reverse cowgirl. To maximize penetration, place a pillow under your hips. So you're laying on the bed or floor, and they're sitting on you, facing away. What's the reason this works? The extra elevation in your hips will make the experience feel deeper to them.

7. The Spork

This is an excellent option as it lets you use your partner's leg to leverage. Have your partner lay on the flooring with one leg stretched straight. Make sure they kneel between their legs and lift the other leg straight until resting against your back. Be sure to hold your leg as you go in the room, and then use it to pull and push into and out.

8. Pole Position

Sit on the other side of a couch, and let your companion sit down and have their legs in the left or right direction rather than straight ahead. This causes the hips to drop a little more than they would in the typical cowgirl posture and will give you the additional penetration you're seeking. You can utilize your hands to raise your hips upwards and downwards, or down, or if in a low position, you can use your foot to lift off the floor to generate momentum.

9. The G-Whiz

This could be the best maximally effective position available. Place your partner on their backs and then pull their knees to their chests and then return so that they lift their hips off the floor. You can then scoot ahead of your partner and then penetrate. If your knees are able, you can sit down next to them, with your knees outwards from yours. This is an excellent position since the hips are elevated, and you can be in control of the strength that your thrusts exert. Practice it on a carpeted flooring or couch to ensure ease of movement.

10. The Flatiron

Your partner should lie on their stomachs with their feet tightly squeezed together. To aid in access, place the pelvis on a cushion. Lie on their backs and come in from behind. Since their hips are at an angle that's more closed than they are, there's more friction on their vaginal walls. The more tightly the legs are squeezed, the more tension and pleasure you'll feel.

11. Flat Doggy Style

Doggy fashion is typically an extremely perceptive position. If your companion has a tiny penis, it might not be feeling that way to you. Change the position of your body by lying flat on the floor and pulling your legs in. This creates a more feeling of fullness. The insertive partner can also spread their partner's butt cheeks apart to help maximize penetration depth. As with all positions, slight tweaks go a long way with this position.

You can pick up your preferred vibrator wand and place it between the legs underneath your body. In this way, you're riding the wand as your partner rides the other way. For those who love the most tension, this sex position for a tiny penis could bring you from zero to orgasm very quickly.

You can experiment with an egg that vibrates in sex if you are in each position. Putting the egg near the cervix will create a more shallow place for your lover's genitals to move. This allows the vagina to appear more full.

12. The Shoulder Holder

One of the most effective positions for a small penis (or strap-on) This move can take the missionary to new heights. Instead of spreading your legs, you can place them on your partner's shoulders. They can be positioned to lean towards your body to give you amazing depth or grip your ankles for extra assistance.

To help maximize penetration depth, you can put a pillow behind the receptive partner's lower back/butt region to tilt their pelvis slightly upward. In this situation, nothing can stand in the way of the partner inserting their way to prevent them from getting as deep as possible. The person inserting must hurry to the closest distance to the receiving partner.

13. Knees To Chest

You should be in yoga's happy-baby position to do this. The receiver lies on their backs, knees pulled up to the chest, and arms wide. The giver is then able to come in from below. The person at the top can utilize their weight to create friction with the clitoris while providing the greatest depth.

This position allows the penis to enter in a very direct and intense way and generates friction with the clitoris, provided that the person on top is well supported. The latter uses Enjoy, an app for sexual well-being. Application for women, you could even incorporate toys with you. Consider something that is small, for example, the finger-vibrating device.

14. The Sideways Ohm

If you give this sexiest position for a tiny penis (or strap-on) an attempt, the person receiving it should be lying on their back while their legs are bent. The receiver then kneels using both knees right behind the receiver's butt and enters from behind. The giver can hold onto the hip to assist with balance or better leverage when thrusting.

The receiver can lift their outer leg to try a different angle if they like

This position is ideal for three reasons concerning intercourse: It expands the vaginal opening to increase friction, allowing the receiver to control the cheeks of the butt as well as the thigh and legs to gain access, and permits the use of an unorthodox angle for entry, resulting in an unusual sensation to the recipient.

This position allows the penis-haver to thrust their full length into the receiver and frees their hands to manipulate butt cheeks and labia to their liking and provide clit access. This position can also be re-adjusted in myriad ways depending on what sensations one is looking for.

15. One Big Leg Up

This sex posture for the small penis requires the penetration partner to lie back on their back, extend one leg, and then place it on their partner's shoulder. The other leg is to be left on the mattress. The person penetrating the other sits on their knees and begins to penetrate with their shins, holding the leg raised with one hand and straight using the other. This posture permits a great deal of flexibility.

If straightening your legs is painful, consider bending the knee slightly. (If you don't have a bed, you could also try this at the table. You can also try these unique chair positions for sex.). The angle at which legs are spread and the height created when elevating one leg permits the penis to penetrate deep. This also implies that both persons can touch other body parts while undergoing penetration and enjoy the experience.

16. Man's Best Friend

Doggy style can work pretty well for a less small size. You must kneel on all fours for the proper posture and let your companion sit on his knees with you or sit behind yourself while kneeling upon the bed. It is important to keep your movements in check in the case of smaller members and doggy-style. Have the guy focus on the extent of his penetration instead of trying to pull the entire way out, as doggy movements could lead to slippage.

17. Seashell

Like the knees-to-chest position, Seashells work well since it permits extremely close PIV contact. Additionally, your partner can grind or make an arc instead of pounding. As you lie in a back position, lift your pelvis forward and pull the legs towards each other so that they are spread into the shape of a V.

Make sure that your partner enters straight down. And as much as you can, reduce the gap between your legs to ensure an even tighter fitting. Based on your movement ability, you can move your legs to the opposite side of the collar bone.

18. Upstanding Citizen

If your bed is a lofty bed, or perhaps a table or countertop that is safe to have sexual relations on, take a sex session with your partner sitting in front of you as you lay back on the surface you prefer. It will help align your pelvis and allow him to have more control. You can also cross your ankles across one shoulder to give him the most comfortable experience.

19. A Woman Bends

The woman sits down on the floor, her back, arms, and torso lying on the ground and her hips slightly raised. The man eases his midsection into position so that his penis will be seen to enter the vagina, and his legs can stretch apart on the opposite side. He then lifts himself with his arms, ensuring no weight over the lady's legs and feet. It is believed that this is particularly effective for stimulating the bottom of your penis.

The penis is more open for a man who has everyday use of a premium penis health creme (health experts suggest Man1 Man Oil, which has been clinically proven to be gentle and safe for the skin). You must find the creme with L-carnitine since this amino acid has neuroprotective properties, which can aid in reducing loss of sensation in the penis, particularly due to rough handling.

20. Splitting Bamboo

This is a great move because it lets you use your partner's leg for leverage. Place your partner on the floor, with one leg straight and the other extended. The ideal position is for the man to sit down between his legs while raising her leg straight up to rest on the shoulder. Hold the leg you're entering, and then use it to push and pull while you push through and out.

21. Pile Driver

If you're trying to find the position with the highest impact, the piling driver position is the best option. You'll need your partner to lay on their back and bring her knees towards her chest to do this. Roll backward until her hips are lifted off the floor. Then you will do a Squat, with your knees moving away from her.

22. Supergirl

Make her lie on her stomach, with her feet tightly squeezed as if she were floating through the sky (hands open in front are not required). Then, you can access her by stepping behind since her hips are in an area that is more closed than open, and more friction will be created on the vaginal walls. The more tightly she squeezes her legs, the greater friction and pleasure you will feel.

7

How Do You Accept Yourself As You Are Regardless Of Size?

A lot of people have difficulty acceptance of their worthiness. They might hear negative comments about their weight or appearance, which could lead people to believe they're not good enough as they are. However, self-acceptance is one of the key ingredients to living an enjoyable and fulfilled life, regardless of your height or size. Learn to be a better person by accepting who you truly are.

Perhaps you've not been giving yourself enough self-worth or dealing with situations that you find hard to take on. Finding the courage to love yourself is a journey that could be a long process; however, it's something that we all have to work on. Accept yourself as well, and your life will become more manageable. Here are some actions you can start to start today:

1. Spend some time with yourself each day. This may be working with your family, friends, or yourself (if required).

2. Write down what you like about yourself and an instance when you were confident about yourself. Many people cannot do this due to their fear of admitting their mistakes and confessing their shortcomings. However, the truth is that all of us have these flaws. Just remember to be proud of your individuality and the thing that distinguishes you.

3. Focus on your strengths and capabilities and not just your weaknesses. Be aware of what you're skilled at, not what you're not skilled at. That's the place where confidence in yourself is born.

4. Develop a healthy self-image. Check at yourself in the mirror and try to identify what

you like about yourself, both from the inside and outside.

5. Be aware of those thoughts that cause you to feel down about yourself. The most challenging issues stem from self-talk and negative thoughts. So, learn to get rid of those negative thoughts by focusing on positive things or taking a deep breath.

6. Try being gentle with yourself and admitting your shortcomings. It's crucial to accept that everyone makes mistakes; therefore, forgive yourself.

7. In the end, join an organization that offers support or an individual who can be there for you when you're looking to discuss your issues with self-acceptance. Writing down your thoughts is a great way to get your thoughts out there. Be careful not to get caught up when you're analyzing your situation. writing or having a conversation with your others can make you feel more

positive about yourself and not get more miserable.

With a little discipline and perseverance, You can begin to accept who you are. If you're feeling down or unhappy about how you treat yourself, Do not hesitate to seek help. Family and friends are too devoted to you to allow you to be a victim.

If you are often staring into your mirror and feel disappointed in your body is time for an overhaul. Finding a way to love your body requires effort and acceptance, but it doesn't need to be complicated! Women who have either plus sizes or skinny, we have many examples of how they have overcome their self-doubt.

The trick is to appreciate every body type as beautiful and unique. Continue reading for a few suggestions to help you accept yourself for the person you are.

- **Loving Your Body Can Mean Loving Your Body**

The first step is that you have to be able to accept the body you are in before accepting it. This involves taking your flaws and imperfections and not the type of self-pity that makes you desire to make changes. When you truly are happy with yourself, it will be simple to accept the way you appear.

However, it is more of a challenge than it is done. If it were as easy, all people would be confident and self-assured before the world. Here are some suggestions to get you started on your journey towards self-love and acceptance.

- **Select Clothes That Make You Feel Beautiful**

Instead of comparing yourself to magazines, begin taking note of women of a similar size.

If you're larger, check out models with larger sizes, and if you're a smaller size, take a look at the celebrities who are happy and proud of their bodies.

Find a dress that you love and feels beautiful and wear it everywhere. Being comfortable in the body that you're in will allow you to accept the look more.

- **Practice Self-Care**

  The body is a beautiful thing and deserves to pamper itself and be pampered, mainly since you are the person who is responsible for it. Enjoy a relaxing pamper day. Relax in long bubble baths with candles and bath bombs, and relax with your most loved films. Give your body a well-deserved massage to make it feel great about itself! It is essential to be gentle with ourselves, as cruelty hurts our bodies.

- **Accept That Everybody Is Unique**

There are a lot of concerns about the physical aesthetic standards, which is a shame. The thing society doesn't consider is the unique beauty of every person. Never compare yourself with other people!

Every shape, size, and body shape is unique and should be praised for its uniqueness. Here are some great ways to accept your body as it is. are:

1. Consider asking your self "what am I grateful for?" before going to bed.
2. Read empowering books.
3. Reward yourself by giving yourself a massage, a bubble bath, or a manicure to reward yourself for the job well done!
4. Attend the opera, ballet, or other high-standard events.

- **Create A List Of All The Things You Appreciate In Your Physique**

Make sure you keep the checklist in mind! This is the first step you must never miss. When you are self-confident and feel you love yourself, it's easy to carry out the actions you take to show self-love. When you start being nice to yourself, it will be easy to begin acceptance of your own body.

- **Affirmations Are An Excellent Method To Begin**

There's no doubt that we've heard of positive affirmations. We've been through them, and I'll admit, there are times when they don't work. However, something can impact our lives - and that is a different way of thinking.

Before you begin your positive affirmations, be sure you've followed the steps in the first place on this list.

One of the most difficult things is proving yourself, even if you don't accept yourself yet!

Make sure you have confidence before writing your goals. Record everything you admire about your body and whenever you doubt yourself, refer to your list.

8

Why Do Girls Prefer A Small Penis?

It has always been a mystery to us whether or not women's size is important. We also sought to understand what women need to fulfill their sexual desires. We need to get rid of another myth. It isn't so much a myth as a perception. The best way to find out is to ask women.

Many men want to know the average size of a woman's penis. When asked, most women responded the same way: "What difference does it make? They're not going to change their size." Men may not be able to change the size of their penis (unless they have enhancements), but they can certainly change their technique, so it doesn't matter.

Although penises may be more practical than beautiful, for straight men, it can be confusing what size penis women like and what makes a good penis. Grooming? Upkeep? Shape? Smoothness? Vascularity?

It is important to know that dimensions are key when it comes down to what makes a beautiful penis. Research suggests that penis girth is more important than most people realize in determining what makes a nice penis.

Whether you were born with a large penis or a smaller one, of average girth or thin, asymmetrical or straight, women are more accepting of what makes a penis appealing than men.

According to one study, women rate overall genital appearance and manicured pubic hair as the most important in determining what makes a beautiful penis. (Credit to the manscaping movement, which is more than hype and marketing. Women did not distinguish between hypospadias-prone men (a condition in which the urethra opening is located on the underside) and normal-looking men (i.e., those with circumcised penises that are conventionally attractive). The information could help to prevent shame and impaired genital perceptions regarding penile appearance.

1. It's All Perfectly Normal

Although the penis is smaller than most penises, it still functions well. They can be masturbated, get erect, and ejaculate all too easily. They are most likely to be stopped by their mental health.

They may be more comfortable with other areas if they have a smaller penis. This is called the desire to please the woman. A tiny penis can make a man very skilled at cunnilingus or with his hands. They want to compensate for their small packages.

2. It Can Feel Smaller When You Are Sexy

Many sex positions allow women to have sex with men with small penises if we forget about the psychological barrier. A surprising fact is that only 20% of women can climax by penetration alone.

Why worry about the size? Positions such as 'X marks spot' or "doggy style" can increase penetration and make it seem longer.

9

Is The Size Of Your Penis Hereditary?

Your genetic makeup is the most important factor in determining your penis size, but other factors can also play a role. Penis size can also be affected by lifestyle, hormones, and other environmental factors.

Some lifestyle changes, such as weight loss, can make your penis appear longer.[1] Also, trimming pubic hair can help improve the appearance of your penis. These adjustments will not alter the actual length of your penis, but they will help you feel more confident.

The size of your penis depends on the combination of genes you have received from your parents, especially the sex chromosomes. The sex chromosomes determine one's biological sexual sex and secondary sexual characteristics, such as rounder hips for females and facial hair for males.

Males have one X chromosome and one Y, while females have two. The "male-determining gene" SRY gene is found on the Y chromosome, passed down from the father. The SRY gene is responsible for the formation of testes and the external and internal male reproductive organs in an embryo.

The Y chromosome is essential for the development of the penis. However, it doesn't necessarily determine its characteristics, such as length, girth, or circumference. This could be more dependent on the X-chromosome, which is only from the mother and has around 900 genes, compared to the estimated 90 genes of the Ychromosome.2

This would explain why siblings have different penis sizes. Each sibling could also be affected by the influence of the X-chromosome, even though they may share the same father.

Penis size can be affected by individual genes, not genes passed down from parents. Penis appearance and length may also be affected by genetic mutations. Genes are the building blocks of a living organism's appearance, behavior, and character. Each gene is passed to a human from one parent. Humans inherit two copies. Numerous genes make up the chromosomes.

Humans have 23 pairs of chromosomes. There are 22 autosomes and one set of sex chromosomes. The sex chromosomes of a person determine their secondary sexual characteristics and biological sex.

Males inherit one of their parents' Y chromosomes and one from their female parent's X chromosomes. Two X chromosomes are passed to females: one from each parent and one from their mother. The genes on the Y chromosome control fertility and male genitalia development.

The Y chromosome determines the penis development and testes. However, it does not determine penis size or girth. These characteristics could be affected by the X chromosome.

The X chromosome contains between 900-1,400 genesTrustedSource, while the Y chromosome only houses about 70-200 genes. This could explain why siblings with identical biological parents have different penis sizes.

Gene mutations can also alter the size and appearance of the penis and other physical characteristics. Although rare, some genetic conditions can influence penis size. These include Kallmann syndrome or Klinefelter syndrome.

The size of the penis depends on many factors, including the person's unique genetics, parental genes, and external factors. We are often asked the most common penis-related question, "Is size genetic?" It's somewhere in the middle of "Does size matter?" "Is length more important than girth?" (For the record, no. That's just my personal preference.

Surprisingly, or perhaps not, the topic of penis sizes has been extensively researched. Scientists have looked at the relationship between penis size and foot size. According to current evidence, genes appear to play a part in one's growth.

It turns out that most of the genetic material for willies comes from their mother, which is a surprising revelation. It is a complex area, but many genes involved in the growth and maintenance of the penis and limbs stem from the X-chromosome. Men have one of the X chromosomes, while women have two. Because boys inherit the X-chromosome from their mother, and selections of that X-chromosome are random, one brother can have large penis genes from one mother's X-chromosomes. In contrast, another brother might have an average-sized penis.

While the father may not impact the child's length, Paduch noted: "If the father has a larger penis, the son will likely have a similar length." Other factors can affect one's size besides mom and dad's genes.

Penis length can be affected by low levels of androgens as the fetus develops. It has also shown that phthalates and other hormone-disrupting chemicals may affect fetal penis growth. This could be due to an alteration in hormone balance in utero.

They can largely control the size of a person's penis. Most members fall within the "average" range. However, it doesn't matter how big you are. However, the number of inches someone can pack does not indicate their sex drive, fertility, or ability to delight a partner.

10

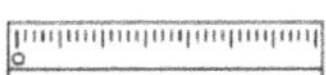

What Determines The Size Of A Penis?

For the first seven weeks of pregnancy, the fetus does not have a penis. Eight weeks after conception, the genitalia begins to develop and differentiate. You'll be able to recall seventh-grade health class. Scientists aren't certain which parent is more influential when it comes penis size. Experts believe that the two X chromosomes of a mother have more influence on a child's penis size than their genetic brothers.

Men with the same father could have the same size penis if the Y-chromosome entirely determined their size. Because size is more likely to be influenced by X chromosomes, one son can inherit penis size genes from both one and the other. One brother might be more well-off than the other.

Although penis size is mostly hereditary, there are healthy interactions between nature and nurture (one's environment). The size of a child's penis can be affected by the mother's use of chemicals like phthalates and drugs such as alcohol. The most pressing medical problem is when a baby's penis is small due to environmental factors.

The most common problem with penis size is when babies don't produce enough testosterone. A micropenis is a shorter penis. Although it can be difficult to tell the difference between a micropenis or a healthy penis, doctors are becoming more adept at diagnosing these conditions early and treating them with hormonal therapy before puberty.

While some may interpret this to mean that testosterone therapy can help them gain a few more inches, Brahmbhatt emphasizes that this is only a treatment that works during childhood and is not recommended for those with micropenis.

Micropenises are rare, and most men don't like their penis size. This dissatisfaction has been associated with low self-esteem and poor sexual health. There is no evidence to suggest that a small penis can affect a man's sexual drive or fertility. Guys, there are ways you can work around a small penis.

Talking about normal, healthy penises with your children is best to prevent self-consciousness. It's important. Children must learn about normal anatomy from their parents. "When they begin to explore, they will probably go to porn. It may help reduce some of their anxiety and stress, but most parents do not.

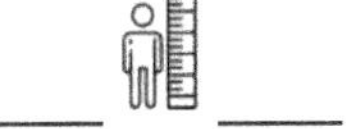

11

Other Factors That Can Affect The Size Of Your Penis

A man's self-image and perception of masculinity and viability are directly linked to the size of his penis. Every man wants a larger and fuller penis. Between the ages 10 and 14, puberty is when the natural growth of the penis occurs. This is when the penis reaches its maximum growth. The penis stops growing in length or girth after 20 years.

A man who finds his penis is too small, insufficient, or asymmetrical loses confidence. A man who has a large penis is more confident and enjoys sex with his partner. While erectile strength, intercourse length, and erectile power are important factors in a happy sex lifestyle, the size of your penis is still a major concern.

The big question is: What factors can affect the size of your penis? There are many things you can do that could negatively impact the size of your penis. You might not be aware of it, and some things can negatively affect the size and shape of your penis. Your hormone levels, diet, stress levels, and smoking status can all affect the size of your penis.

- **Hormone Levels**

    Testosterone, the hormone that causes puberty in men and gives them their male characteristics, is responsible. It stimulates facial hair growth, deepens the voice, and aids in the growth of the penis; between the ages of 12 and 18, penis size increases. If testosterone levels are lower in men during puberty, it could impact the size of the penis. Some men might try to stimulate additional growth with anabolic steroids and exogenous testosterone.

It is not a good idea to do this independently without consulting a doctor. This can cause serious damage to the prostate and testes. The studies that looked at men who took these supplements to enhance their performance found no significant increase in penis size.

The average growth was only one centimeter. This is because steroids increase blood volume. As testosterone levels decline, men over 50 may experience a decrease in penis size. The average man will see a half-inch decrease in his penis size as he gets older.

- **Smoking And Tobacco Use**

Smoking can decrease the size of an erect genital tract. According to this book, smoking has the same effect on the heart as on the penis. Smoking can reduce blood flow and cause a decrease in elastin production, which is what allows men to erect.

- **Diet**

Your diet can directly affect your penis size. A healthy diet can indirectly control your penis size in puberty and after that. Healthy eating habits are essential for proper blood flow. This is vital to the growth and credibility of your penis.

You should eat lots of vegetables and fruits rich in antioxidants to maintain a healthy penis. Antioxidants fight free radicals, protect the body, and keep blood vessels healthy. Antioxidants are also known to increase blood vessel strength. Vasodilators are particularly important because they keep blood vessels dilation muscles open and improve blood flow. Vegetables such as tomatoes, sweet potatoes, tuna, eggs, milk, and milk, are excellent sources of vasodilators.

To reduce the possibility of fat deposits accumulating and clogging the penis arteries, men should eat diets high in fiber and low fat. High-quality foods include avocados, strawberries, raspberries, and beets.

- **Stress**

Stress can lead to a reduction in the size of the penis. As you know, stress can lead to a variety of diseases. Constant stress can cause problems in blood circulation and blood flow. Insufficient blood flow to the penis can cause problems with sexual health.

Stress and anxiety can affect the brain's functioning and communication with the body systems. Erectile dysfunction is when the brain does not send the correct signals to the penis. Excessive stress at work and in personal life can lead to erectile dysfunction. Stress does not refer to the stress of working in an office. Many life events can cause stress.

Relationship problems can cause excessive stress that can negatively impact your sex life. You must be aware of your stress levels if you want to have a healthy penis and enjoy your sex life as much as you can.

Men should be concerned about their penesis size. It's a key indicator of how men feel about their bodies. 4 out of 5 men thought their penis was too small. Penile enhancement was considered by 45% of men.

Every day, I see men in my office who feel negatively about a small penis. Penile enhancement procedures get excellent results. It is important to avoid things that can negatively impact your penis size.

- **Environment**

Penis size may be affected by environmental pollutants such as pesticides, plasticizers, and other chemicals. These chemicals could act as endocrine disruptors. They can also impact gene expression and gene expression.

- **Nutrition**

Malnutrition during pregnancy and throughout your life can impact hormones and cause problems with growth and development. Malnutrition during adolescence can also relay the trusted Source of normal puberty.

Individuals who experience delayed puberty usually get up in the end. However, delayed puberty symptoms include a smaller penis or testicles.

12

Is Surgery To Increase The Size Of Your Penis Worth It?

It is very rare to need penis-enlargement surgery. Men who have a congenital disability or an injury that affects the function of their penises should not need surgery.

Some surgeons offer cosmetic penis enhancement using various techniques. However, this procedure is controversial, and some consider it harmful and unnecessary. These procedures should not be considered routine. Unfortunately, there are not enough studies on penis-enlargement surgery to provide a clear picture of the risks and benefits.

To lengthen the penis, the most common surgical procedure is to cut the suspensory ligament. This connects the penis to the pubic bone. The penis will appear longer if cut because more of this ligament is hanging down.

However, a cut to the suspensory ligament can make an erect penis unstable. Sometimes, the suspensory ligament can be severed with additional procedures such as removing excess fat from the pubic bone.

To make the penis thicker, you will need to take fat from the fleshy part of your body and inject it into the penis shaft. Although the results may not be satisfactory, some of the injected fat might be absorbed by the body. This can cause penile curvature, asymmetry, and an irregularly shaped penis.

Grafting tissue onto your penis shaft is another way to increase width. These procedures have not been proven safe or effective. They can also affect your ability to erect and potency.

Penis enlargement can include a variety of procedures that aim to increase the length and girth of your penis. Most people undergo the process for cosmetic reasons.

Penis enlargement surgery can work in certain cases. However, it is not guaranteed to succeed, and there are some risks. The majority of people who choose to have the surgery are healthy and functioning, so it is cosmetic. These cases can make them cost-prohibitive for some people.

13

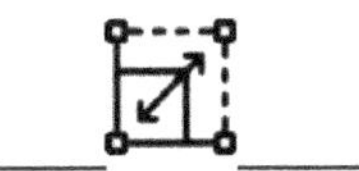

What is Penis Enlargement Surgery, And How Can It Help?

Penis enlargement surgery aims to expand the length and girth of your penis. The surgery may include the insertion or transfer of fat cells and skin transplants to increase the size of the penis. Cosmetic surgery can also create the illusion of a longer penis.

Penis enlargement is rarely necessary. Surgery is only required if there is a micropenis condition. A penis measuring 7.5 cm or less when stretched is known as micropenis. Surgery is not necessary for a penis that functions well enough to allow sexual intercourse and urination.

A 2020 review found that most people seeking treatment for their penis size are within the normal functioning range.

What is the procedure?

There are many options for penis enlargement surgery. Each one has its method.

- **Implants Made Of Silicone**

    This surgery involves the incision of a crescent-shaped, medical-grade silicone piece under the penile skin. It is used to increase the length and width of the penis.

    The FDA has approved the Penuma penis enlargement procedure for commercial use following the 510(k).

    First, a surgeon will make an incision above and then insert a silicone slip into the shaft of your penis. The surgeon will then shape the silicone implant to fit the size and shape.

- **Fat Transfer**

A fat transfer procedure involves the removal of fat cells from the body to inject them into the shaft. This is done by inciting your penis and injecting purified fat into these areas.

- **Suspensory Ligament Division**

This ligament attaches the penis to the pubic bone. This ligament connects the penis to the pubic bone.torontocircumcision4

The surgeon will cut the ligament and move the skin from the abdomen to where it meets the shaft of your penis. This may cause the flaccid penis to hang lower, but it doesn't make it larger.

The surgeon may recommend other procedures, including removing excess fat from the area around the penis. While it may make your penis appear larger than it is, this does not alter its length.

- **Many People Yearn For Larger Penises**

> Dick size is the topic of brotherly banter and bullying, a source for pride and shame, and the inspiration for cultural phenomena with phrases such as "big dick energy" and "gray sweatpants thirst," which are tossed around a lot.

Like for lips and butts, modern medicine has created a variety of methods for people to grow larger-by increasing their length and girth through surgery. Niro Sivathasan, a cosmetic surgeon, says that surgical penile enlargement is still a secret.

Penile enlargement surgery has always remained one thing that not many men would talk about, but it was readily available information. Many men who want their penis enlarged believe they are too small. Unfortunately, clinics don't seem to notice this.

This should be a problem for private surgeons. It is wrong at every level." Most of these surgeries are done in the private sector, and they are often very expensive. The penile extension is similar to a hernia repair and costs PS3,000 on NHS. The penile extension can cost up to PS40,000. Overall treatment outcomes were poor, with low satisfaction rates and a significant risk of major complications, including penile shortening, penile deformity, and erectile dysfunction.

Men who want to increase their penises need structured counseling. If the patient wishes to have a longer penis after the counseling, they can be counseled first to use penis extenders. They can be used regularly to stretch the penis. Although these devices are less expensive than surgery and last for a shorter time, the researchers doubt their effectiveness.

"We believe that men should only be fully informed about the technical issues that may occur, have been told all the facts, and have gone through a complete psychological assessment. Counseling was effective in helping men understand their penis and not undergo any further treatment." It is better to learn facts about yourself than to undergo surgery.

The surgery may include inserting or transferring fat cells and skin transplants to increase the penis size. Cosmetic surgery can also create the illusion of a longer penis.

Penis enlargement is rarely necessary. According to the Urology Care Foundation, surgery is only required if there is a micropenis condition. A penis measuring 7.5 cm or less when stretched is known as micropenis.

Surgery is not required for a penis that functions well enough to allow sexual intercourse and urination. A 2020 review found that most people seeking treatment for their penis size are within the normal functioning range.

It is not something to take lightly. This can have severe consequences for your health and well-being. Sometimes, however, surgery is the only option to fix an embarrassing problem or make a cosmetic adjustment. It is important to remember that surgery can be more expensive than initially thought. There may be procedures that are very affordable or cost-free.

A hymenoplasty is an operation that can correct a genital condition, such as difficulty having intercourse or having children. This operation repairs the hymen and any damage it has done. Women will experience soreness, discomfort during sex, and problems taking birth control pills if they don't have surgery. This is due to the scar tissue in their hymen. It is a simple procedure that takes less than a week to complete and requires no stitches.

Another option is to consider a hymenoplasty if your doctor discourages you from having surgery on your penis. The surgeon will simply remove the affected area. The surgeon will also be capable of removing scar tissue from previous operations, whether they were performed before or after your birth.

Transwomen who desire a natural appearance and are happy with surgery results will be pleased to hear that it is highly recommended.

Due to the scar tissue that develops over time, some people may need a hymenoplasty multiple times. This is particularly true for sexually active people. Sometimes, scar tissue can cause pain when intercourse is continued or in conjunction with other activities. If you continue to engage in sexual activity, it can cause tiny tears.

If it occasionally happens and does not cause any severe harm, you can use ice packs to relieve the pain and wait for your pain medication to kick in before returning to normal. Sometimes scar tissue can cause pain in the bowel or full bladder. This is particularly true for women with urinary tract infections.

Sometimes the condition can be genetic. It is best to talk to your doctor about whether it would be better to have the procedure performed young or wait until you reach adulthood. If you feel that surgery to remove your penis is too costly, it might be worth considering hymenoplasty. It is less expensive and causes less lasting effects than other surgical procedures. The surgery also offers more than aesthetic benefits.

You should not limit your choices to those listed. Surgery can be dangerous, and there may be other risks. Before you undergo surgery, ask yourself these questions: What are the risks? What are the advantages? Are all options considered? Do I need to do this? Do I regret it? Will I be able to handle the after-effects of anesthesia/surgery/pain?

This is crucial if you decide whether it is a good option. You will not get the complete story from your doctor and may not receive accurate answers.

You should also avoid seeking out foreign medical professionals. You should verify the credentials of any medical professionals you seek out from other countries. Many procedures and practices are unsafe or ineffective in countries other than those you live in. However, it is okay to use them in your country.

Some doctors in certain parts of the world may even offer surgery to boys when they are young or without explaining what is happening. Some surgeons may simply remove a portion of the penis to stop it from growing and potentially causing injury to the boy as an adult. If the penis is abnormal or deformed, they might perform a penectomy or circumcision.

A doctor who performs this type of surgery will not guarantee the boy's ability to have an erection as an adult. They are legally required to inform you about what they do and allow you to make an informed decision. It would include whether it is safe and the potential side effects or risks. You can still get confused if you don't have the answers you need.

Many doctors are still not familiar with penile surgery. Trans men may wish to eliminate their penis and genitals. Some doctors will perform these operations and offer consultations on safe procedures. While they understand their controversial nature, they also realize that surgery may be necessary if a child is born with something similar or later develops.

Others disagree. Some doctors believe that hormones determine a person's gender identity. One thing is sure, although the surgery may be more costly or more complex than other surgeries, it is still worth the effort. Be wary of surgeons that charge lower than the others. You should be wary of surgeons who charge less than others.

Although penile surgery is still a relatively new procedure, many things can be done to improve the methods used. Some operations will permit transgender men and women to be their preferred gender without the need for hormone therapy or other invasive procedures that can prove risky.

14

⸻ ❧ ⸻

Conclusion

You can take some actions to make it through life with modest manhood. You can increase your confidence by being authentic while remaining positive and not letting your masculinity determine your character. Many like-minded people share your passions and will support your efforts.

In addition, you can consult with experts or men who have experienced similar challenges and have learned to overcome these challenges. Conquering any obstacle is to admit that you've got one. Once you've recognized the problem and accepted it, you can begin working to resolve the issue.

Get help from a professional if you aren't comfortable talking about your personal life with family or friends. Get help from a professional. It is essential to realize that there are many ways to achieve success in life, no matter the size of your body.

Success can be achieved by making goals and doing your best or through making connections and networking. Whatever your age, keep in mind that you're competent in whatever you want to accomplish. So don't be afraid to try new things and be the person you'd like to be. But most importantly, never quit on yourself!

What is more complex than making it through life with the size of a man? Most men will answer an unquestionably yes. The culture has taught us to think that having a small size is a negative issue and that we should take action to combat it. The reality is that there are plenty of successful men in the world who have had to struggle with unassuming manhood.

Some things will help you be successful in your career while having the smallest of manhood. First, don't be scared to seek out assistance. Remember that you're not on your own, and many can relate to the struggles you're experiencing. Thirdly, make sure you are taking care of yourself physically and mentally. Do not let your manhood define you. Remain confident in your self-worth and the things you can do.